# EATING HEALTHY

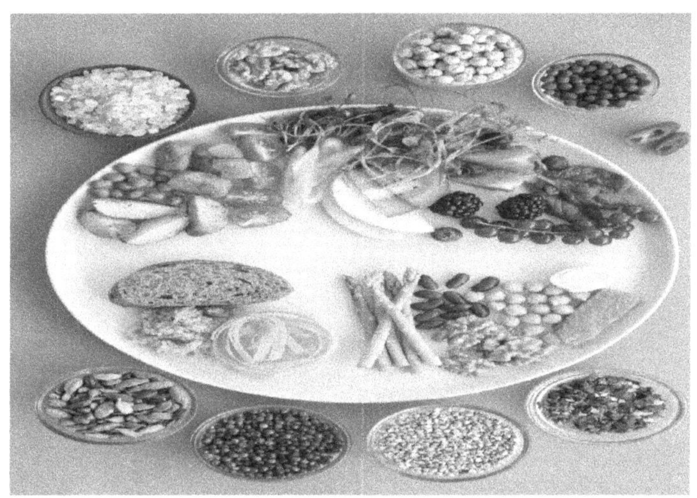

*Experience a Healthier You: Eat Your Way to Better Living*

# DR WILLIAM WHITE

# COPYRIGHT

# Disclaimer

The writer has strived to be essentially as precise and complete as conceivable in the formation of this report, despite the way that he warrants or addresses never that the items inside are exact because of the quickly changing nature of the Web.

While all endeavors have been made to confirm data given in this distribution, the writer takes care of blunders, oversights, or opposite understanding of the topic thus. Any apparent affronts of explicit people, people groups, or associations are accidental.

In down-to-earth guidance books, similar to whatever else throughout everyday life, there are no certifications of payment made. Perusers are advised to answer on their own judgment about their singular conditions to appropriately act.

This book isn't expected for use as a wellspring of lawful, business, bookkeeping, or monetary guidance. All perusers are educated to look for administrations with respect to skilled experts in lawful, business, bookkeeping, and money fields.

You are urged to print this book for simple perusal.

# Table of contents

Foreword

In basic terms, the body has two altogether different and complex frameworks of fuel-creating sources. As energy is imperative to the actual presence of human action and endurance the two energy styles rely upon one another for help. This book shows you what food sources give you the most energy.

It happens so regularly - we resolve to happen with a well-being and actual workout regime with zing and logical much exhibit as well; but in the main seven-day stretch of going into the arrangement, all that subsides.

Can anyone explain why we don't stay with the eating routine plans, the early daytime running plans, and the actual activity designs that we make?

Furthermore, how may we guarantee we continue onward with these plans, for the good of our own and for the people that are subject to us?

Is it true that you are eating just to fulfill your craving or to make your taste buds blissful? Or on the other hand, would you say you are eating to assume better control over your life? In this digital book, we perceive how you can make your life substantially more ideal essentially by causing a direct that you toward eat accurately.

Practicing good eating habits

# CHAPTER 1

## The Nuts and Bolts

Energy is required for different capabilities like the support of development, day-to-day exercises, work out, and numerous different developments or capabilities that are frequently underestimated. These are divided among the two energy frameworks.

In this day and age, only here and there do any well-being and wellness plans work. What's the justification for their disturbing pace of disappointment?

The world is significantly less restorative than it was twenty years prior. A lot of this is credited to the changed food habits for people.

The essential and first to-be-utilized energy framework is the vigorous framework. This framework involves oxygen for the capability of the muscles and requests a considerable amount from the general body framework.

This request ordinarily builds the rate and profundity of breathing and blood supply basically due to the related expansion in the pulse.

At the point when the body requires more energy which can't be met because of the raised requirement for more oxygen then the body framework consequently changed to the anaerobic energy framework. This framework can deliver energy without the need to utilize oxygen.

This energy is produced through the appropriate or addressed utilization of food sources. The food varieties ate direct the sorts of energy levels every individual is fit for delivering.

Muscle weakness generally happens when all the energy sources are depleted which can be credited to various reasons; the most convincing one relies upon the sorts of food varieties eaten.

There are a few classes of food varieties that produce different helpful components for the human body framework and taking note of the ones that make or improve the energy-creating sources is certainly valuable to be aware of. Subsequently, this information ought to assist the person with picking the right sorts of food varieties.

The high-impact framework works by separating the carbs, unsaturated fats, and amino acids in the food sources eaten while the anaerobic framework lets energy out of the food sources put away in the body, ordinarily during extreme movement sessions.

In the event that we catch wind of the disappointment of diets or exercise center plans surrounding us, generally, it isn't their issue. Regularly the issue of the people began with much upheaval about going through these plans, informing every one of their associates and collaborators, and afterward didn't submit to those projects.

The people who leave the activity or consume fewer calories midway don't see the benefits, normally, and everyone faults the arrangement.

What the world necessities these days are definitely not new well-being or workout schedule or an eating routine, yet it requires inspiration. It needs the right kind of mentality to completely finish anything that plans they have decided as far as possible.

In the event that they can do that, a large portion of the medical problems that are connected with the way of life circumstances will become outdated. Furthermore, we don't need to visit the sides of the earth to find this inspiration. The inspiration lies here, inside us; we essentially have to look through it out and use it.

One age prior, people wouldn't fantasize about getting anything low-quality food they might set up to take care of their countenances. These days, that's what we do so nonchalantly. "I'm ravenous" generally signifies "I need a burger or a wiener, possibly with chips as an afterthought and some cola." And, "I'm on a careful nutritional plan" signifies "I'm on a synthetically ridden pill which will overcome my yearning and deny my collection of nutrients." It's really no big surprise that we are confronting so many medical problems today.

Our well-being is a mark of what we consume. The sorry condition that we're living in is certainly not a singular issue; it's a worldwide issue. The world all in all is eating mistakenly. Six in every ten people in the US is overweight, and the number will be eight in every ten people when we hit 2015.

Is it safe to say that we are really pondering this? We aren't. Indeed, even as you're concentrating on this Book, you probably have a bundle of chips as an afterthought. Do you have any idea that what you spent on that bundle, which is filling your stomach with the absolute most harmful synthetic compounds known to mankind, could rather have taken care of a thin young person in Ruanda?

However, it's not just about being magnanimous. It's about us as well. Indeed, we must be self-centered. With such shocking well-being figures, would we confirm or deny that we are setting out toward destruction? We're certainly not eating right. Whatever overabundance stuff that brings - stoutness and the different chronic sickness afterward - we must be ready for it.

So the following time you see that a program has fizzled or is getting a great deal of analysis, recollect that the analysis isn't presumably in light of the fact that the program remains in peril. Generally speaking, it is on the grounds that individuals started with incredible expectations and afterward didn't follow the program as they ought to have.

# CHAPTER 2

## The Manner in which You Ponder Food

The most urgent thing that you really want to keep your well-being and workout schedule alive - considerably more vital than a teacher or a specialist - is your own thought process.

You are not entirely set in stone to examine what is happening. Thus, you're overweight and are seeing pushing off a couple of pounds. No rec center teacher from any spot on the planet will help you in the event that you don't go to satisfactory lengths to have the right eating regimen and adhere to your standard activity.

Regardless of whether you're debilitated and are taking a gander at treatment, no doctor will help in the event that is not entirely set in stone in following the treatment stage, whether it's taking the medicine at the right time or going without certain food sources.

We have wandered terribly with our dietary patterns so far. Except if we assess the situation and assume control over issues, matters won't improve.

The number 1 thing is mindfulness. We need to realize what food varieties are right for us and what aren't. We need to return to preparing and appreciating what the supplements are that your body genuinely needs and in what sum.

Then, at that point, we need to fabricate a dietary routine for us as well as our friends and family so we eat better. We need to eliminate every one of the food varieties that are antagonistic - the sugars, the fats, the starches, we don't genuinely need them - and integrate food varieties that might help our well-being.

This sounds excessively long-winded, I get it. However, that is the main relief we have. Assuming we keep crunching on Oreos, we're never going to improve.

Yet, there's trust. Trust lies in the way that there are a lot of food sources out there that are basically essentially as delicious as those terrible unhealthy foods yet we have hardly any familiarity with them.

These are the food varieties that we have barely any familiarity with yet, we probably could do without them or we don't have the foggiest idea how to fix them, yet a solid cookbook might help you in grasping grouped fascinating ways to sound cooking.

Indeed, even with a similar kind of diet you eat, you can invoke a few truly tasty solid dishes. Indeed, it's all a lot conceivable. You can change your dietary patterns to a major degree, while simultaneously taking care of your sense of taste.

The truth of the matter is that the weight reduction industry is mindful in a truly huge manner of this destruction of the created human race. They need to continue to sell their Atkinses and Jenny Craigs and Zones and Medifasts and hence, the media never let you know how we may, in all actuality, assume control over things.

They show us marvelous before-after photos of an individual with a foot-long sub and afterward the very fellow with 6-pack abs and let us know that the eating routine made that conceivable.

In any case, the truth of the matter is, if we somehow managed to get our heads together, we may effectively do that as well, without burning through 1000s of dollars on those eating regimens. Also, what do we need to do?

2 general things:-

**Control what we consume.**

**Enjoy actual effort**.

Presently, is that an excessive amount to achieve? Don't we owe that to our body that has served us so well for such a long time? Don't we owe that to ourselves and our friends and family?

# CHAPTER 3:

## Honey and Entire Grains

Throughout the long term, honey has been demonstrated to be the one supporting power behind the energy circle. Helping the human body in different regions it is first still unparalleled in its energy-delivering substance. Honey is nature's most normal energy supporter. It likewise goes about as a viable invulnerability framework developer while giving the regular solution for a large group of differed sicknesses as well.

Energy is vital to the smooth streaming normal of the day-to-day existence pattern of any individual. Along these lines finding energy sources that are both predictable and solid is essential to staying in shape and cheerful.

### A Decent Pair

The regular advantages of honey have been broadly recognized and acknowledged. Other than its extraordinary taste, honey is likewise a characteristic wellspring of carbs, which is an energy producer for helping execution, perseverance, and decreasing degrees of muscle exhaustion.

This is valuable for competitors. The sugar content in the honey assists with assuming a forestalling exhaustion during exercise meetings and furthermore during instructional courses for sports devotees. These sugar make-ups are isolated into glucose and fructose and capabilities in various however praising ways.

The glucose content in the honey is by and large consumed at a quicker rate and radiates a prompt jolt of energy while the fructose works at a more slow speed for more manageable and delayed energy. With regards to tending to glucose levels in the body framework, honey has been known to assist with keeping the levels genuinely consistent.

As honey is a lovely food item and it's normal in its structure, devouring it's anything but an undeniably challenging activity. Individuals of any age are by and large very able to consume honey in any of its going with structures. It's even well-known among youngsters.

The energy delivered from consuming a limited quantity of honey every day assists youngsters with adapting to the actual types of day-to-day school exercises furthermore, sports responsibilities. For grown-ups too consuming a day-to-day little portion of honey can go far in keeping the energy levels at their best during a requesting day at work.

Making sandwiches with honey went with different fillings is one approach to making a wonderful tidbit. Applying honey on a newly toasted cut of bread is likewise a welcome breakfast elective. Adding honey to drinks as opposed to utilizing sugar is certainly energized.

The vast majority today needs a handy solution for their energy-helping requirements and this normally comes in the undesirable types of sports beverages, espresso, and refined carbs like sugar and keeping in mind that bread.

However these produce the ideal elevated energy levels, it ought to be noticed that this energy is genuinely fleeting and the sleepiness that follows is generally more intensely felt. Consequently picking to consume some type of entire grains isn't just a superior other option but at the same time is a lot better.

Entire grains give the energy that arrives in a more complicated structure that separates over a more drawn-out timeframe. This then makes the stage for supporting the energy levels for longer periods.

Due to its more complicated make up the entire grains accompany a variety of valuable components like minerals, nutrients, phytonutrients, and fiber which are likewise wealthy in fiber.

Adding the entire grain fixings is any dish that generally finishes the flavor or improves it through and through. Entire grains can the different structures like wheat, oat, grain, maize, earthy colored rice, faro, spelt, emmer, einkorn, rye, millet, buckwheat, and some more.

These can then be made into different items like entire wheat flour, entire wheat bread, entire wheat pasta, moved oats or oat groats, triticale flour, popcorn, and teff flour.

The advantages of consuming entire grains reliably can assist with diminishing the gamble of coronary illness, lower cholesterol levels safeguard against many kinds of disease, and aid weight the board. Entire grains ought not to be mistaken for their lesser and more refined "cousin". However refined grains have a few advantages it is in every case better to settle for general grain options

# CHAPTER 4:

## Nuts and Lean Meat

Nuts are a significant wellspring of supplements for both human and creature utilization. Being wealthy in an entire host of essential supplements it tends to be eaten in its crude structure, cooked, or as an added substance to currently prior dishes. Though nuts are characterized as a hard-shelled organic product, there are numerous different food varieties that are remembered for the nut family.

Various sorts of meats by and large add to different flavors, but the best kind is the one with however much lean meat content as could reasonably be expected. It's an undisputed reality that meats that contain a lot of fat are a culinary treat without a doubt however for well-being purposes carving out the opportunity to comprehend the advantages of consuming lean meats is extremely savvy to be sure.

## Great Proteins and Oils

It is presently considered normal information that nuts extraordinarily help in holding a lot of diseases within proper limits or from happening by any means. For example, nuts have been known to have the option to keep the chance of coronary heart infections showing, in any event, for those entire come from a long queue of relatives with this issue.

Consuming nuts like almonds and pecans have been known to bring down serum cholesterol fixations inside the body framework. Nuts are additionally enthusiastically suggested for those people experiencing insulin opposition issues like diabetics.

Going nuts rather than unhealthy food to control desires is additionally another better other option. Containing fundamental unsaturated fats is likewise one more addition to the moment when it comes to picking nuts as a better other option. Since nuts are sound and can be consumed in their crude structure, it is likewise one more added benefit to keeping these around and convenient as tidbits.

Almonds are frequently used to standardize blood lipids on account of their gradual process attributes, which help to keep the glucose levels reliably solid. Rich in a changed measure of various supplements the almond is a famously added substance to the lifeless eating routine of most Mediterranean individuals.

The Brazil nut is additionally another nutritious nut that accompanies its own arrangement of advantages when consumed with some restraint. Noted for its omega-3 unsaturated fat substance, the Brazil nut is likewise a decent wellspring of calcium.

Cashew nut is one more extremely famous nut that is many times consumed as a salted tidbit. Anyway, it would be a lot better food item without the expansion of salt, as it is now a seriously tasty nut all alone. In certain regions of the planet, these nuts are made into oils.

The choice interaction ought to be finished with just the right amount of information as relying entirely upon what the unaided eye sees isn't sufficient. For the most, lean meats got from hamburger cuts ought to incorporate round, throw, sirloin, and tenderloin, while the cuts from pork or sheep would comprise tenderloin, flank hacks, and leg. The most slender pieces of the poultry would be the bosom region without the skin.

However there are many reasons individuals wipe out meat from their day-to-day diet, there is no proof to show that this is a positive or negative decision nor would it be a good idea for it to be trailed by all.

Anyway, the significant highlight note here is the decision of the kinds of meats that would make the utilization solid and this would commonly mean meats with a lesser measure of fat substance. However white meat is in no way, shape, or form ailing in fat substance, it is by examination considerably less in fat substance than red meats.

The dietary benefit of consuming lean meats is very broad and adjusted. Lean meats have a by and large higher and cleaner content of protein which is a vital contributing variable to key primary and practical advancement of each and every cell food and development.

Lean meats are likewise a decent wellspring of fundamental amino acids, especially sulfur amino acids. When contrasted with the stomach-related rates the proteins in meats work quicker than the ones contained in the beans and the entire wheat range.

Lean meat is likewise a decent wellspring of iron. Since the lack of iron is moderate it is frequently not distinguished until a later stage when paleness has been created.

# CHAPTER 5:

## The Advantages

Here is all the thought process you'd expect to keep practicing good eating habits.

We should quickly dive into the subject.

Benefits

## You Get Healthier

We could entire assortment of books about the well-being benefits of eating accurately yet it wouldn't exactly cover what benefits really exist. The main benefit is that you gain control over your weight.

By eating accurately, you in like manner verify that your metabolic capabilities - most prominently your safe framework and your gastrointestinal framework - continue to work accurately. You're moreover shielded from arranged constant illnesses, right from cardiovascular infections like coronary vein sickness and hypertension to diabetes.

## Savvier

Practicing good eating habits implies you spend substantially less. Your bills at the general stores descend radically and you don't dive farther into charge card obligation assuming that is now an issue with you. Furthermore, you save an enormous group on all the medical services costs you'd require in the event that any issue surfaces in light of your food-gorging habits.

## Fewer Poisons in Your Body

A lot of food varieties these days are poisonous in light of the engineered synthetic compounds present in them. While you're endeavoring to eat accurately, you are substantially less liable to get these poisons into your body as one of the fundamental authoritative opinions of eating accurately is that you shouldn't eat anything that is man-made.

What's more, assuming you eat less, you'll in like manner have the option to diminish indecencies like smoking and liquor abuse. A glass of brew is practically inseparable from a night out with the young men. On the off chance that you eat less, you won't need the lager also. Essentially, you won't need that (at least one) required smoke that you will more often than not have after every feast.

## More Actual Way of life

At the point when you eat better, you'll observe that you can take care of your responsibilities in a greatly improved manner. You can practice more, travel more, play more, work more, and accordingly make your life more useful.

That definitely beats being a fat good-for-nothing and relaxing around on the lounge chair the entire day, right? You can likewise be more associated with your companions and friends and family and that definitely advances your life.

## Great Public activity

Disregard fat fetishism, people who are overweight don't look engaging. There are areas of strength for a no about weight on some unacceptable spots of the body. On the off chance that you're attempting to find an accomplice, your fat may in a real sense disrupt the general flow. Not just that, people who have zero control over their dietary patterns and subsequently their weight are peered downward on by society as being people who have zero control over their essential inclinations.

This kind of brain science exists, however not many people will talk about it. At the point when you eat accurately, you'll find that such issues vanish.

## Conclusion

There are a ton of well-known slims down available these days, yet a large portion of them are undesirable and periodically even risky. This will clear up how to eat a solid, adjusted diet forever and avoid unfortunate weight control plans.

Learn the number of calories your body expects to work consistently.

This number might differ fiercely, contingent upon your digestion and how genuinely dynamic you are. In the event that you're the kind of person who lays on ten hammers out plainly smelling a cut of pizza, then, at that point, your consistent caloric admission should remain roughly 2000 calories for men, and 1500 calories for ladies.

Your weight similarly has an impact in that: More calories are proper for normally greater people and fewer calories for humbler people. In the event that you're the kind of person who can eat without acquiring a pound, or you're genuinely dynamic, you could wish to build your everyday caloric admission by 1000-2000 calories, a piece less for ladies.

Try not to fear greasy food varieties.

You need to devour fat from food sources for your body to accurately run. In any case, choosing the right kinds of fats: Most creature fats and a couple of vegetable oils are high in the kind of fats that raise your LDL cholesterol levels; the foul cholesterol is urgent.

Not quite the same as prevalent thinking, gobbling cholesterol doesn't unavoidably rise how much cholesterol is in your body. In the event that you give your body the right devices, it will flush additional cholesterol from your body. Those instruments are monounsaturated unsaturated fats, which you should attempt to routinely consume. Food varieties that are wealthy in monounsaturated unsaturated fats are olive oil, nuts, fish oil, and arranged seed oils.

**Eat a lot of the right carbs.**

You need to eat food sources high in carbs since they're your body's main wellspring of energy. Try to choose the right carbs. Basic carbs like sugar and refined flour are immediately consumed by the body's gastrointestinal framework.

This initiates a kind of carb over-burden, and your body discharges immense measures of insulin to fight the over-burden. Not exclusively is the abundance of insulin terrible for your heart, but it energizes weight gain. Eat a lot of carbs, yet consume carbs that are gradually processed by the body, for example, entire grain flour, veggies, oats, and natural grains.

**Eat greater dinners right off the bat in the day**.

Your digestion decelerates around the finish of the night and is less effective at processing food varieties. That implies a greater amount of the power put away in the food will be stacked away as fat and your body will not retain as numerous supplements from the feast. Take a stab at eating a medium-sized feast for breakfast, a major feast for lunch, and a little feast for supper. Even better, endeavor to consume 4-6 little dinners over the run of your day.

**Give yourself a cheat feast**.

Cheating doesn't mean pigging out on every one of some unacceptable food varieties one time each week; it infers in a portion of food you genuinely love one time each week. Two or three cuts of pizza on Sundays, or a colossal cut of twofold chocolate cake on Saturdays. This cheat feast will assist you with staying with the adjustment of diet, and in a couple of ways it's truly great for your body. Unique events, similar to birthday celebrations in the family, consider cheat dinners.

**Get the habit for eating gradually**.

It will fulfill you with fewer calories and will thwart indulging and corpulence with every one of its ramifications.

**Drink a lot of H2O.**

It causes you to feel more conscious and invigorated, ponders for your skin, and causes you to feel fuller so you end up eating less! Chopping down pop and supplanting it with water will do wonders for you.

www.ingramcontent.com/pod-product-compliance
Lightning Source LLC
Chambersburg PA
CBHW071559270726
48657CB00027B/2322